M

Learning ment

Introduction:

Why you need to read the whole story

I have and been involved in direct patient care and performed knee replacements for over thirty-five years. During this time, I became aware of two absolutes. The first is that physicians assume patients have an unrealistic level of medical knowledge. The second is that patients rarely ask or are intimidated regarding questions about their medical condition.

I became aware of this issue when I was a fellow in training for reconstructive knee surgery. I had just completed a final examination with the senior physician on a patient needing knee surgery. It was a rather straight forward knee issue involving the need for ligament repair.

As the last patient of the day, the senior physician was not rushed to go to the next patient and had given a lengthy explanation of the problem to the patient. I suspected the discussion and explanation was as much to educate me in the fine art of physician-patient interactions as it was to inform the patient. This new patient consultation occurred without his family members being present,(his request), during the visit.

They waited patiently in the waiting room. The face-to-face explanation about the condition and the needed intervention took about 15 minutes. During the discussion with the physician, the patent was given an educational booklet related to his problems. There were pictures drawn in the booklet that pointed to the problem and areas were highlighted which related to his knee. No aspect of the surgery or the medical condition seemed to have been ignored in the explanation to the patient.

I was impressed by the completeness and thoroughness of the information presented by physician. In fact, I was somewhat suspicious that the time spent with this patient was aimed more to impress me than the thoroughness of the doctor.

After the discussion with the physician, the patient nodded in agreement that he understood the problem with his knee. He had decided to have reconstructive surgery and proceeded to schedule the surgery.

The day ended and I headed to the elevator to leave. Entering the elevator, I found myself with the same patient who had just been seen for knee surgery. This new patient apparently did not remember or recognize me. He was relating to his family what he understood was his medical problem and necessary treatment . The family members asked what was going on with his knee. The patient responded, “Something is wrong, I’m not certain what it is, but it needs surgery.” A length medical discussion about his condition had been reduced to a single simplistic sentence.

This new patient had no idea or understanding about his condition. He did understand it was serious and needed surgery. The problem was the physician was speaking in a language that was foreign to him And that is the crux of the problem. Physicians assume the patient understands the language of medicine. The patient is either intimidated, embarrassed, or reluctant to admit that there is a clear absence of any real understanding of what is being discussed. This language barrier, resulting in confusion and a lack of understanding with patients is common.

The medical language used by doctors is a foreign tongue. Physicians use words in front of patients and assume everyone knows the language being used. Words such as “patent vessel, "tracheal atresia” or "dehiscence" are included in a talk about risks of surgery. It is assumed that everyone understands what is being said. A doctor will state to the patient, “Your knee has an effusion" . It is expected that you understand he is referring to the fluid in the knee joint.

The physician is not being arrogant. It occurs because doctors interact mainly with other physicians. The terms and words become so commonly used and accepted in these professional interactions that they become part of the everyday vocabulary. It is assumed by the doctor that everyone understands the language of medicine. This language barrier causes a problem and results in the patient not understanding what is being said. If the patient reluctantly asks for more information or clarification, the answer often increases the confusion.

I once asked a patient to flex the injured knee. The patient looked at me without moving. It was a simple request. It took me a moment to appreciate that the patient didn't understand the word "flex". I had assumed that everyone understood the term referred to bending the knee. To this patient, I could have been speaking in Russian.

Medical terminology confusion is even more obvious in the informed consent. The patient signs this form before surgery. It states that there is a complete understanding of what is about to happen. Terminology and descriptions are used which are so complex that few patients understand what they are signing. Patients sign consents for a "transsphenoidal hypophysectomy". It is doubtful if the person signing had ever seen those words or understood the implications of the consent.

A major Boston Hospital once considered a simplified consent. The new consent would state that medicine was imperfect, mistakes might happen, and severe complications might occur. All treatments would be based on the best knowledge and science. Everyone understood that description. It was simple and straightforward. And, of course, it was never put into practice.

The lack of detail was felt to put the hospital at risk The simplicity of the document was based on the premise no patient could ever say they didn't understand what they were reading and signing. Some physicians try to explain medical problems to patients by using explanations that are too simple. By making it too basic, the patient gets a distorted understanding of the problem.

I have heard patients tell me they got an injection of "oil" into the knee for lubrication. There is no such product. The physician tried to explain to the patient that the product being injected was a lubricant, like oil. The product given actually increases the synovial fluid viscosity (thickness). However, by making it easy to understand, wrong information was given.

I have written this story about Molly, a woman that develops knee pain It is written to be read in one sitting. The story will take the reader through the onset of symptoms, the treatment of knee pain and a decision to have joint replacement surgery.

When Molly's story is over, the reader should be able to empathize with the character of this book. This is a not a science book. There are no diagrams, picture, graphs or drawings. This is a story that will provide the reader with a thorough and detailed knowledge of knee pain, arthritis and joint surgery. It is meant as a gateway of information.

Visualizing the story will provide longer lasting understanding of the medical issues than simply looking at diagrams. If more information is needed, this story will be the groundwork for any future reading. Molly is not meant to be an example of every type of person who will have surgery. She will encounter problems and ask questions. She will get frustrated and have typical roadblocks to treatment. Her experience will give information helpful to both sexes, all ages, and all body types.

Why a story? When a patient seeks information about knee surgery the result is typically a book or pamphlet with a combination of pictures and diagrams. In this modern age of technology, a lack of images or video links makes written information seem old fashioned. Pictures are sometimes hard to understand. They are often so simplified as to be cartoonish. Or they are so detailed that they don't help. Patients leave confused after an office visit and often toss the pamphlets in the garbage as they head from the physician's office to their car.

Memory and understanding are enhanced through visual imagery. Reading or hearing a story may provide a greater understanding and the perception. Consider the following. Look at the number "21232986" for two seconds and try to memorize it. Then tomorrow morning try to repeat it from memory. However, suppose you were told in a story that an important number was the boiling point of water, the freezing point of water, and your body temperature. The next day, 212- 32-98.6, would be easy to recite. Visual imagery improves memory and understanding of a problem.

Molly's journey will be a story of gaining awareness about injury and treatment of the knee. Her tale does not require any knowledge or understanding of knee pain. There is no need for an understanding of the complex issues of knee anatomy. It is a tale about her experiences.

Through this parable, the reader will learn about the treatment of the painful knee and the need for knee replacement surgery.

Chapter 1

Molly has knee pain

As Molly walked to pick up her 14-year-old daughter Abby from the soccer field, she noticed some pain on the inside of her left knee. This was worse than the pain she had been experiencing on occasion the previous six months. It was sharp, stabbing, it took her breath away. She wanted it to go away and it was sticking around like a shard of glass in her knee. With a slight grimace and limp, she soldiered on.

Molly did not appreciate that this pain was due to a problem that would start her on a path where there was only one outcome. She was beginning a new journey. One that she never expected nor could have anticipated. She was unprepared and had no knowledge of how to prepare for the end result. And, unlike her previous adventures, this one ended with a knee replacement.

Her daughter, Abby, jumped into the passenger side of her new Silver Chevy Tahoe. The SUV involved spending more money than she and her husband Homer had wanted to spend. The decision was made easier when she rationalized that their lives had changed. They now had to deal with a gaggle of girls going to soccer games and the three family dogs who went with them on local trips. They needed extra room for equipment, people, and animals.

Placing her left foot on the running board, she swung into the driver's seat. This time the pain was sharper and made her grimace. Abby noticed the change in her mother's smile. "You OK?" Abby questioned with mild concern. "Mommy's fine, honey." The standard answer to resolve any teenage angst.

On the way home, Molly found that keeping her knee bent with her shoe on the footrest next to the brake did not help the pain. She had to keep moving the position of her leg to help the discomfort. Bent or straight, the pain was still there.

As they drove home, she glanced up as they passed the Galactic Fitness gym. She had joined it six months ago to shed the middle age weight gain that seemed to be happening to everyone she knew. Joining the gym was an attempt to keep her weight stable.

Between her job as a financial advisor and taking care of the family, exercise was not in the daily planner. Unfortunately, her work as a financial advisor was more sitting than activity. She had developed a habit of munching food while driving due to the stresses at work. The 15 pounds gained had turned to 20 pounds. On her five-foot five-inch frame, she felt the size difference.

To make matters worse, when she did go to the gym, the slow jogging and walking she tried on the treadmill always seem to cause her left knee to ache. The elliptical was hard to manage and she still had the pain. She tried the knee machine. She figured if she sat in a chair and straightened her knee with weights on her ankle, there wouldn't be knee pain.

Unfortunately, this made the pain worse. Even walking on the treadmill caused her knee to hurt. Using the chair while lifting leg weights caused her knee to hurt. Her body was telling her not to exercise. And Molly dutifully followed her bodies advice.

On getting home her limp was a little worse. That annoying pain that at times seemed to come and go wouldn't go away.

She limped into the kitchen and was greeted by flurry of tails. Three black rescue dogs ran to her expecting treats. Each dog weighed no more than 30 lbs. so there was no concern about them hurting her knee. Still, Molly instinctively turned to protect her left side. Homer greeted her in the kitchen and saw her limp to the dog treats on the counter. After the biscuits had been gulped down, Molly opened the cabinet and found her bottle of naproxen. She had been told that the over-the-counter medication was the same as the prescription drug, just a smaller dosage. She swallowed two naproxen sodium tablets, an amount equal to 440 mg which was still less than a prescription Naproxen at 500mg . She followed it with a swig of water and handed out three more biscuits to the frolicking hoard of happy four-legged creatures.

She had taken two naproxen tablets that morning and her knee still hurt. Molly figured it would be ok to take more than the maximum of three a day, even though there was a warning on the bottle. She was in pain. She hoped the naproxen would work.

She had switched to the naproxen when the three 200mg ibuprofen tablets she had been taking three times a day proved ineffective. And that dosage of ibuprofen was more than recommended by the warning on the bottle. Tylenol didn't help and she needed to have a functioning knee. There were too many things going on to let this slow her down.

It was after dinner that the swelling occurred. Molly noticed that she had trouble bending her knee. It was now painful and looked like a melon. She elevated her foot on a chair. She had heard that ice would make swelling go away. What was needed was sleep and rest. The knee would be better in the morning. So, off to bed, ice pack on knee, pillow under the knee which seemed to help, and an antacid for her stomach which was starting to bother her. "More like someone punched me in the stomach" she thought out loud, "than real pain. Probably nothing a few antacid tablet won't cure."

Chapter 2

Time to See the Doctor

The following morning, Molly felt exhausted. Her knee had bothered her throughout the night. Every time she fell asleep, she would move her knee and the pain would wake her up. The night seemed to last forever. She looked over at Homer. Despite her tossing and turning, he was sleeping like a log. He never seemed to have any trouble catching his needed rest. He never had any pains or problems that kept him up and he never gained weight.

Molly was both envious and angry that his life seemed so much easier. As she got out of bed, she found her knee wouldn't bend or straighten and the swelling seemed to have gotten worse. It wouldn't straighten out enough for her to stand up without leaning to the side. When she did put weight on it, it felt as if it might buckle and give way. “I really don’t have time for this," she thought. She grabbed a fairly beat-up pair of crutches from the closet. A leftover souvenir that Abby was given after an ankle sprain last year. They were a little short, even after adjusting the length, and the rubber tip was worn down. With one crutch under her left arm, it did help support her left leg.

As Molly limped to the kitchen the dogs followed her and she let them out the back door to the fenced in yard to enjoy the morning dew. Abby, the oldest, came in and dutifully took the dog dishes and filled them with their morning mixture of canned food, freeze dried toppers and nutritional supplements. Abby was careful to make certain that the dogs got the best nutritional support. Although Abby would only eat a defrosted waffle for breakfast, the dogs ate a fully balanced meal.

Molly sat down, opened her laptop, and did a quick web search for orthopaedic specialists. When Abby had injured her ankle, the local sports clinic had provided care. The clinic didn't look like the place to go for a painful knee when there was no injury. It appeared to be more of a place for the injured high schooler. Plus, she wanted a specialist who would treat her adult injury and get her going as quickly as possible.

Googling "orthopaedic knee pain" she got a listing of over 100 sites. It seemed that everyone was treating knee pain. The listing included therapists, chiropractors, holistic treatment centers, lawyers looking for clients who had treatment issues, sports clinics and arthritis centers.

Trying to narrow it down, she added, "physician knee pain specialist". This did get her predominantly a list of physicians and clinics that had physician associations. But, as before, the list was overwhelming. Everyone seemed to be willing to treat knee pain. And they all stated and promised that they were the best. "Time to call Jason." she mumbled under her breath. He worked with her as a co-worker and also worked with her at her job giving financial advice.

Last year Jason hurt his knee while squatting down to fix the brakes on his not so vintage Mustang. He saw a physician and ended up having a simple surgery that got him back to near normal in just a few weeks. Jason had commented that the doctor seemed to be understanding and did not rush into surgery. They had tried several treatments and options until all non-surgical interventions had been exhausted. After his surgery, his recover was quick and there did not seem to be any lingering issues. A call to Jason at the office got her the name of Dr. Stephen Katz. The office was a 25-mile drive. She was assured that it was worth the travel to get a good specialist.

Molly rationalized the distance by telling herself that Homer drove twice that far to get an expert to fix his classic Austin Healey 3000. “ A good mechanic is worth the trip!" he would declare. And Molly felt getting good treatment for her knee was as important as getting a qualified mechanic for an aging 60-year-old British car. Plus, the car repairs were not covered by insurance.

After a phone call to the doctor's office, she was told that there were no openings that day. The receptionist promised to leave a message with the doctor in case there might be a spot at the end of the day.

Molly tried to play the pity card. She said she was miserable and could barely walk. That got her a response that if it was that bad, she should go to the Emergency Room. Molly responded she it wasn't all that bad and she would wait by the phone for a call back.

While she waited, she did try some other offices just to get options. She found out two things. The first was that every physician office has an automated telephone system that must be sold by the same company. The electronic voice at the other end of the phone always started, “If this is an emergency, call 911 and go to the hospital”.

Apparently, no doctor wants to see an acutely ill person.

The second realization was that every physician in the area was booked. The next office opening was over 2-3 weeks away. The sympathetic receptionists did suggest the family doctor or the ER. Getting an appointment and seeing the doctor was sometimes over a month away. Several offices had a physician assistant and she could see the PA and have an earlier evaluation. Molly felt that the PA was more for a minor problem. Her problem was serious and needed help.

Just as she got shot down after her fifth call trying to get an appointment, her cell phone rang and she was told that Dr. Katz could see her today at 4:30 PM. That would just about kill the entire day. Regardless, she took the appointment and called her office to let them know she would not be in. Missing one day wouldn't be that bad. She hadn't taken a day off in a year. Jason could cover for some of the work and some could be done on her laptop while she sat at the kitchen table.

Chewing two Tylenol, then two naproxen for the pain, Molly propped her knee up on a chair, put a pillow under it, and applied a Ziplock bag with ice. Abby gave her a quick hug and scooted off to get to school with a breakfast biscuit in her hand.

While sipping her coffee and working, Homer came in from his office where he was working on a research proposal to submit to the Army. Working as an industrial psychologist meant submitting offers for a project and hoping it would be accepted. It did allow Homer to have flexible hours if he was in between jobs.

Seeing Molly looking miserable , Homer offered to go with her and do the driving. She gladly accepted as her knee was getting stiff and all those pills were making her stomach hurt. While thanking Homer for his kindness, the physician's office called and asked for insurance information. She hadn't thought that the medical insurance they carried might not be accepted by the doctor. There were HMOs, PPOS and then open plans. Her coverage was accepted. She was informed that a co pay of fifty dollars would be required at the time of treatment.

Chapter 3

The Office Visit

Molly and Homer pulled up to the office entrance at a spot marked for patient drop off/handicapped parking. For the first time in her life Molly appreciated the easy accessibility of the spot to the entrance. Using her crutches to walk to the door which opened automatically, Homer parked the car in an open spot almost 25 yards away.

She waited for him at the entrance on a bench that was conveniently located near the elevator. Checking the sign near the elevator, the medical offices were on the third floor. Therapy was on the second and the first floor seemed to be an administrative/billing section. They pushed the button for the third floor and exited into an open waiting area filled with over 15 people in chairs. Many of the people were obviously family members of patients, there for emotional support. Molly glanced at the crutches, walkers and canes propped against most of the chairs, waiting to be used.

Walking to the front desk, she signed in. A young receptionist asked for her insurance card and photo ID. She then gave her a clip board and asked that she answer all the questions and sign it before the exam.

Molly took the papers and sat in a chair next to Homer. She looked at the five double sided pages to be answered and wondered how much of this information was really needed. Many of the questions were about how her injury occurred. Was this a work injury? Was a lawyer involved? Did this involve a motor vehicle accident? Molly smiled realizing that the office was trying to determine which patients might have a legal issue and involved a lawyer.

A long form authorizing the release of medical records for insurance purposes and billing needed signatures. Also, she filled out a HIPAA acknowledgement and a listing of who was authorized to see her records. The Health Insurance Portability and Accountability Act was intended to protect patient information. Her own experience with HIPAA following her daughter's ankle injury showed there was confusion and misunderstanding of the requirements by most physicians and offices. Molly struggled to have her family doctor get a copy of Abby's ankle MRI from the first treating clinic because Molly had not faxed, ("who uses faxes?") her signature and authorized release to the MRI unit. She later learned that the needed fax was unnecessary. The law states that patient care will not be impeded or treatment delayed. However, the MRI receptionist did not understand the law and was following a protocol that was set up by someone else who did not understand the guidelines.

The medical history looked like something she had filled out dozens of times before. She denied major injuries, surgeries, or medical conditions. She checked no to a list of almost 30 illness or conditions. She had no allergies. Codeine made her sick and some antibiotics made her queasy. These weren't allergies, just side effects. She knew there was a difference and didn't want to prevent a treatment and the use of a possibly less effective medication because of a mild side effect. She did indicate the nausea under "reactions," not "allergy".

She handed back the information and dutifully took her seat. After only 15 minutes, they called her name. She went with Homer through a door and into a corridor with 10 exam rooms. Some were open with patients being escorted to different areas, some were empty. Obviously, they had a busy clinic and more than one physician was treating multiple patients at a time.

Changing into her shorts she was told to bring, she sat on an examining table while

Homer took a comfortable chair in the corner. After only a few moments, a pleasant curly haired 20 something assistant came in and sat at a computer console. The name badge indicated her name was Tiffany.

After smiling at Molly, she entered some information, took Molly's blood pressure and checked the height and weight. Asking about any current medications, Molly said she took nothing purposefully neglecting to mention over the counter medicines. Tiffany recorded she was on no medications, unaware of the use of the ibuprofen and naproxen.

The assistant left and a pleasant woman opened the door. She had a radiology detection badge and told her that she would take a series of x-rays before the doctor saw her. "Hi, I'm Judy and I'll be taking your x-rays." Everyone seemed so pleasant and happy. Molly followed her to a small room where the x-ray technician efficiently took a set of x-rays of both her left and right knees. Two were with her standing and putting weight on the leg and two were while lying on the x-ray table. Molly asked why she had to stand and get both knees x-rayed. The technician told her that often subtle changes of damage are more apparent when the joint is loaded with the person's own body weight. Also, if there is a subtle finding, comparing the normal to the injured knee helps determine what might be a normal variation.

Molly returned to the exam room and checked her messages. No major issues at work. Jason was helping solve any problems. Either that, or he was simply not letting them get to her. He knew she was concerned about her knee.

The physician walked in, mid height, 50's, with mainly dark brown hair that was starting to gray. His hair was wavy but trimmed. No white coat, just a dark gray suit jacket with white shirt and blue tie. He wore round gold rim glasses that reminded Molly of a 1960's style. Looking like someone who tried hard to maintain his fitness, he sat down on a stool near the corner.

He took a clip board and looked at her through his gold rimmed glasses and introduced himself. “I'm Dr. Katz.” he said in an upbeat manner, “and this is your...?”. “My husband, Homer.” Molly answered. “Never assume anything,” Dr. Katz said with a smile. “You would be surprised how often it’s not the husband. It could be a friend, relative, son, or partner. Making the wrong guess can be a big mistake.”

A quick review of the problem and the history confirmed that the knee pain had been sporadic for six months with the severe issue for only 1-2 days. He had her lay down comfortably on the table and reassured her he would not cause her any discomfort. Asking where the area of greatest pain, she pointed to the inner aspect of her left knee, just below the kneecap area.

He commented on the swelling and then gently bent her knee about ¼ of the way back. He gently touched the area and she confirmed the discomfort. His fingers rubbed over the inside and outside of the knee. After straightening it out, he pressed on the swollen area at the top and sides and seemed to be evaluating the amount of the swelling.

He referred to the knee swelling as an effusion. A new term for Molly. She was to hear that word many times in the next several weeks. An effusion was fluid in the joint from internal irritation. It was almost never a good sign.

After professionally pulling on her knee in several ways and pressing on her kneecap in an effort to check how easily it moved, she was told to bend and straighten her knee . This was hard due to the swelling. As Dr. Katz put his hand on the kneecap, he apparently was trying to evaluate for noises or grinding sensations. “Hmmm, “ he muttered. “Kind of noisy. “

Another word was used to record the noisy knee. She found out it was called crepitus. And, like an effusion, that grinding noise called crepitus was also rarely a good finding.

Turning to the computer monitor, he pushed some buttons and the x-rays that had been taken appeared on the screen. "Well," he said as he turned the monitor so both she and Homer could see it, "The right knee looks great! That left knee has some significant issues."

Chapter 4

Molly Learns Anatomy

Over the next 15 minutes, Dr. Katz gave Molly a description and explanation of the problem. He told her that it was not unusual to have only occasional pain with a sudden onset of discomfort that would send a person to the hospital or doctor's office. She learned that there are often conditions that are relatively unnoticed or symptomatic. Then, a minor twist, like getting out of a car, or jamming the leg on a stairway, can cause everything to fall apart. Just as a glass with a crack may shatter with a mild tap, a minor trauma to the knee can suddenly cause a hidden problem to become symptomatic. The condition had been there for a while but was only now becoming an issue.

And her condition was arthritis. Dr. Katz described the knee joint as having two large bones that come together and form a complex joint What allows us to bend the knee, twist, jump and climb without the knee falling apart is that the two bony surfaces have ligaments that hold them in alignment. These ligaments are just like tension ropes on a tent. They keep the bones correctly positioned.

There are four ligaments. There are ligaments on both sides of the knee, and internal ligaments that control from and back motion.

These four ropes or ligaments stabilize the knee. If they are injured, like in a soccer injury, the knee is unstable. Molly had heard of the condition of an anterior cruciate ligament tear that was common in football players. Homer's brother Mark had such an injury playing soccer. He ended up needing it repaired in surgery.

Dr. Katz added that all of Molly's ligaments are fine. Molly listened as she was told that the two bones of the knee joint form a surface that is curved to allow motion. One bone is concave or curved out like a ball. It is the top bone or femur. It is the largest joint in the body. The other is convex or curved inward like a socket. That is the tibia. It is smaller and a somewhat less curved.

The femur, the top bone, look like two upside down scoops of ice cream. The tibia, the lower bone, has two shallow cups to accommodate the two surfaces of the femur. As Molly pictured the knee joint, she was told that nature doesn't want bones to touch.

To stop the bones from rubbing on each other, bones have a covering called cartilage. "It like the laminate on your countertop that covers the wood base, or the Teflon on your frying pan," Dr. Katz explained. "When healthy, it is smooth like ice and shiny. It is only about ¼ inch thick. It's tough and should last your lifetime. When two cartilage surfaces touch, it is more slippery than ice skates on wet ice." "But" Molly wondered, "why do people say they have a torn cartilage if the surface is cartilage? How can the surface cartilage be torn?"

Dr. Katz told her that In order to help distribute the weight between these two curved surfaces there is a meniscus. This is shaped and works like an O ring or washer between two parts coming together. If the top and bottom surfaces have any offset or don't meet perfectly, this cartilage acts just like the washer in a faucet. It solves the problem of two surfaces that aren't seating perfectly by deforming and helping distribute the weight. She visualized trying to carry a heavy box on her head. If you put a round donut of rubber between the box and your head, it will distribute the weight. That would protect your head from too much weight at a single point.

This round rubber ring is the meniscus. It was the meniscus that was torn when people said they had a cartilage tear. Dr. Katz stated this was a common misunderstanding. She now understood that the common perception of a torn cartilage is actually a tear of the meniscus. The meniscus is a form of fibrocartilage. However, fibrocartilage or the stuff that makes the meniscus has nothing to do with the surface cartilage. The cartilage that covers bone surface is hyaline cartilage and it the loss of hyaline cartilage that causes arthritis.

Dr. Katz described what arthritis was and how it looked. "When the cartilage layer thins or becomes injured, the underlying bone can be exposed. And the exposure of the bone makes the surfaces rough. They lose the slippery effect of the shiny joint surface and start to grind away. As they grind away there is pain and swelling. "

Molly learned that cartilage of the knee will not regrow or heal. The joint surface, or the hyaline cartilage that you have as a young adult, has to last you for life. Once it is damaged or thins out, it will never return to normal. In the knee, there is no recovery from the loss of hyaline cartilage. There is no second chance after a cartilage injury.

Surfaces continue to deteriorate and wear over time with more exposed bone. The effect is like taking sandpaper to the Teflon pan. As the joint continues to wear, the pain may progress slowly, or like in Molly's case, be sudden in onset.

Looking at her x-rays, Molly could see that the bone surfaces on her left knee were closer together than on the right knee. The cartilage which is invisible on x-ray and keeps the bones separated was missing in her left knee. Looking at the x-ray of both knees, the left knee bones were touching. On the right knee the clear space was obvious. The bones were almost 3/8ths of an inch apart.

Molly understood what was going on. The shiny surface of the knee that protects the bones was wearing out. This surface would not regrow or come back. And the surface was worn out enough that bones were starting to touch and grind away. She had developed bone on bone arthritis. No wonder her knee hurt.

Chapter 5

What Caused This?

Molly looked at Homer with an unhappy and miserable look. “What caused this?” she asked She looked at Dr. Katz and told him that she had been an active basketball player and cross-country runner in high school. Mollies want to know if she had worn out her knee due to sports. She was thinking that she should restrict Abby’s sports to prevent future arthritis.

Dr. Katz told her that there was no evidence that simply running or playing in sports caused arthritis. It was believed that in some people there may be an old trauma to the knee. It might be minor, yet the injury could be the reason for the arthritis. It might take twenty or thirty years before the injury causes a problem. Molly recalled dozens of times she had fallen or injured her knee and had not had it evaluated. There were too many injuries as an active person to seek attention for every little bump.

Dr. Katz added that not all injuries cause later problems. Many athletes have injuries and do not develop issues. "Lots of arthritis is thought to be idiopathic and simply occurs over time", Dr. Katz told her. That meant there was no obvious reason or understanding why it occurred. "This type of arthritis from aging was called degenerative or aging arthritis. Sometimes referred to in a more common term of osteoarthritis.

It was simply due to a premature loss of cartilage. It had nothing to do with activity. It is no more related to activity than baldness is due to washing and combing your hair every day. "

Molly found out that the term arthritis simply means joint pain. It could be from infection, called septic arthritis, or from crystals in the knee and called gouty arthritis. At times, the body may attack itself and destroy the joint due to an autoimmune condition. That was rheumatoid arthritis. There were even arthritic conditions associated with skin lesions called psoriatic arthritis. Hers was the most common type of arthritis. It was degenerative or osteoarthritis. Possibly due to a decade's old injury, or possibly from just bad luck and genetics. The effect was the same. The cartilage cells of the knee were injured and were dying. She told Dr. Katz that her sister and mother had no knee issues. Her father had knee pain towards the end of his life., He had died quickly from a heart attack and was never treated for the pain. Dr. Katz assured her that a family history sometimes is found with arthritis. However, it was more common for this type of arthritis to be from injury or just from unknown reasons. “ I have gained some weight” she offered in the hope that maybe weight loss would make the problem go away.

Dr. Katz felt that her weight gain was not the reason for the arthritis. Although weight gain can cause arthritis, it needs to be excessive. Typically, weight gains of over 50 pounds are needed for someone her height to have a significant impact. And, that kind of arthritis from weight gain usually shows similar damage in both knees.

"So essentially my knee is wearing out." Molly expressed with some worry. "We don't know why, maybe an old injury. We'll probably never know." She looked at Homer for some support and reassurance. He looked upset. He stood and put his arm around her to offer support. "What do we do now?" he asked as he gave Molly a gentle squeeze with his hand.

Chapter 6

It's Time to Start Treatment

"OK, so what do we do now? How do we treat it and cure it?" Homer turned to Dr. Katz. "What's the next step to get rid of her pain?"

"Well, one doesn't cure arthritis," Dr. Katz stated. " One treats the symptoms. If the pain and discomfort is better, then everyone is happy. Each person has a different need. Only if the pain continues to interfere with the quality of life and activity, do you ramp up the treatments. My suggestion is to start with something simple. Evaluate the improvement and determine the next step based on how Molly feels she is doing. " Dr. Katz turned to Molly. "Right now, your knee is so swollen and painful that you need crutches. I recommend that I drain your knee of the fluid and inject it with some medicine to help the pain and swelling. That would give you some immediate relief. I would then also add a prescription arthritis medication to take orally. This will help the swelling and the let's have you start some therapy for your knee. "

Molly was curious about what the injection would be and was it dangerous. Dr. Katz told her it was a form of a steroid. It was called dexamethasone. It would stop the swelling and pain. He would combine it with a small amount of a type of Novocain to help any discomfort from the needle. " I thought steroids in the knee could cause arthritis. Don't they mess up with your blood sugar and make you gain weight? I'm definitely not going to want that problem." Molly added, " And if it works, is it permanent or just a quick fix?"

Steroids in the knee, she was told, are highly effective at stopping the knees reaction to the arthritis. It effectively calmed the knee down. As long as the shots are not given more than three times per year, they would not cause damage to the joint. Most of the problems with steroids injected into the knee occur when people receive injections on a weekly or monthly basis. Also, the shots should only be done if there is significant improvement that lasts for at least eight weeks, and then no more than three times per year.

"Think of the steroid like nose spray for a runny nose. It should make you feel better and hopefully, the reason for the runny nose will be better before the medicine wears off." Dr. Katz then explained that the steroids in the knee should have no effect on any other part or her body or her metabolism. “Yes, it was true,” Dr. Katz added, “steroids have side effects. It's the oral pills that are absorbed into the body that are the major culprit, not injections. Although there may be a sugar change in some people after a knee injection, that was mainly in diabetics and the sugar change is temporary and returns to normal in just a few hours. “

He also added that there are two types of steroids. The kind that body builders take were anabolic steroids. They do nothing for inflammation. She was going to get a catabolic steroid. It wouldn't build muscle but would help inflammation.

"And the medicine and therapy? What good will that do?" she questioned. " My stomach is a mess from all the naproxen and ibuprofen I've been taking. I belong to a gym, why do I need therapy?"

Dr. Katz responded, "All great questions and concerns. I should have checked your chart more closely. I didn't see any indication that you were taking any other medicines. Are there any other medicines I should know about?"

"Well," Molly responded, "they are all over the counter medications. You don't need a prescription. I figured they were safe and I didn't need to mention them. I don't take anything other than the ones for my knee pain."

Dr. Katz admonished her by saying even non prescriptions arthritis pills like naproxen and ibuprofen can have side effects. Considering the amount and frequency Molly was taking, she was actually exceeding the prescription level of the same medication. This was a common problem that Dr. Katz said. It often led to bleeding ulcers. People didn't realize that just because a medicine doesn't require a prescription, it can be taken in large and frequent doses to equal the prescription form. And, it will have consequences and side effects as bad as any prescription drug. . He felt it would be prudent to place her on a medicine for her stomach to prevent any future issue and to carefully monitor for any other problems associated with the medications.

Regarding how to exercise and do therapy, Molly was told that many people just don't know how to exercise the knee in a safe way. In fact, many of the exercise machines at the gym could make her knee worse. The treadmill and the knee extension machine may actually increase her discomfort, which was exactly what had happened to her at the gym. So, therapy would show her the correct way to work out and strengthen her knee. This would allow the muscles to absorb the shock of walking and maybe make her knee feel better.

Molly agreed to the plan. Step one was drain and inject the knee. Then, some therapy for the knee.

Chapter 7

Draining the knee

Homer came over and provided Molly with emotional support while the Doctor told Tiffany to get the necessary items for the injection. Molly was told to lie down and for comfort they placed a pillow under her painful left knee.

While the assistant was getting the syringes, the Doctor proceeded to wipe her knee off with a special cloth that had a solution to kill bacteria. "It's not alcohol," Dr. Katz told her. "That's not strong enough. We use chlorhexidine. That kills just about everything. The risk of infection in this procedure is about one in 5000. Even with those low risks, it's important to always take every precaution."

Wiping her knee in increasingly large circles, he used two different wipes and disposed of them after use. Then, after putting on gloves, the assistant placed the three syringes on the table. Molly gulped. "Don't worry, I won't feel a thing, " Dr. Katz quipped. His humor was lost on her as she was clenching her fists in anticipation of pain.

After first using a "freezing" spray she felt a small burning sensation on the outside of her left knee at the middle of the knee cap. "That's the numbing medicine. That should be the worst of it!" Dr. Katz muttered as he reached for the next syringe. She felt a pressure and then a strange feeling in her knee. Like a balloon was deflating. "I'm getting a lot of fluid out. Is there any pain?" he asked.

Molly refused to look. Surprisingly, she felt no pain, just a little discomfort. Then, after draining out the fluid, Dr. Katz removed the syringe leaving the needle in place and attached the syringe with the steroid medicine on the hub of the needle that was still in her knee. He injected the milky medicine and pulled this syringe and needle out. He immediately placed a sterile pad on the injection site. “All done!” he exclaimed. “That wasn’t too bad, was it?”

Surprisingly, Molly had to begrudgingly admit it wasn’t bad at all. Much less discomfort than she expected. Now, her knee felt much better. She gingerly bent her knee. The motion had returned and the pain was better. “Wow, does it always work that fast? I thought steroids took days to work," Molly asked.

“That’s the effect of the lidocaine and removal of the fluid. The steroids take a day to work. The pain relief from removal of the fluid and the numbing medicine is almost immediate. There may be some rebound discomfort when the lidocaine wears off, but it shouldn’t be too bad?” he added.

Holding up the vial that held the fluid from her knee, Dr. Katz critically looked at it. “Clear yellow,” he announced. “Consistent with arthritis. No evidence of anything else such as crystals, infection or rheumatoid disease." He then put a strip of paper called a dipstick in the fluid. "Checking for white cells to make certain there is no infection. That can always be a cause of a pain" he explained. After a few moments, he looked at the stick and confirmed there were no white cells or any chance of infection. "It's quite a simple test. Easier and quicker than sending off for cultures, and almost 95% confirmatory of an absence of infection at a fraction of the cost."

Molly was now feeling somewhat better without the fluid in the knee. Homer asked what was next on the plan. Always the analytical scientist, Homer wanted to know the logical and step like progression of treatment. His mild OCD required everything to be laid out in a plan.

Dr. Katz then went through a detailed description of the standard treatments for the type of arthritis Molly was experiencing and causing her pain. Following the aspiration or draining of the fluid from her knee, therapy and the medications would be started. Hopefully, there would be a good response and that might be the short-term solution and treatment. If the knee continued to hurt or the swelling returned, then an MRI would be needed along and a trial of a different medicine or different types of injections. If everything failed and the pain was continuing, a knee surgery might be considered.

Dr. Katz assured Homer and Molly, surgery would only be option if Molly were still in pain and had tried every avenue of treatment over a period of several months.

"OK," Homer muttered. This explanation provided a short-term balm to his anxiety and concerns. He was happy that Dr. Katz was not a knife happy surgeon. He had heard to many stories of surgery being scheduled after only one visit to a doctor.

"Tell me why we don't get the MRI now." Homer wondered. He was told that the only way to make a diagnosis was with an MRI. Everyone he knew was getting them every time their knee was in pain.

Dr. Katz carefully explained why Molly didn't need an MRI at this time. MRIs were typically used for diagnostic dilemmas where the cause of the condition was in doubt or unknown. MRIs could confirm the diagnosis. In some cases, an MRI is helpful with clarifying the extent of the problem and any associated pathologies that might be hindering recovery. If surgery is being planned, it might show the location of nerves, vessels and conditions that would be important to the surgeon.

Molly's problem was obvious on the x-ray and was arthritis. The x-ray gave a clear and unequivocal explanation of what was causing the problem. Only if the pain continued or the condition changed would an MRI be needed. It might give insight and understanding of the extent of the arthritis. It would be a reasonable test if the medicine and cortisone didn't help. If Molly felt better, than the MRI would not add information that would change the treatment.

"My friend told me that his doctor got an MRI right away and injected his knee with an oil or gel shot when he had arthritis." Homer continued, " I would think that it would be best to get lots of information now and try something that sounds like it might be better than cortisone. I hear about the gel shots on TV and read about them in a magazine on the airplane. Don't they cure arthritis."

"Homer," Molly said in a tone she used when trying to let Homer know he was starting to be annoying, "let's see how this does with the medicine and therapy. No need to do unnecessary tests and do more shots. Let Dr. Katz treat it in a way he feels best. "

"That's all right," Dr. Katz responded in a tone that was surprisingly pleasant and understanding despite Homer's confronting tone. Dr. Katz had obviously had family members like Homer in his office many times. “Many people get MRIs on the first visit. As I said, if surgery is urgently needed, an MRI does help. However, MRIs are over utilized and unnecessary if the diagnosis is obvious. The initial treatment will not change. The cost of all the MRIs that are done because patients insist on them adds significantly to the healthcare costs without providing any treatment benefit. And, if you don’t get better,” Dr. Katz said turning to Molly, “an MRI will be ordered.”

He then grabbed a small, padded stool on rollers and sat down. Boosting the seat height up to a comfortable level using a side lever, he rolled the stool back and leaned against the wall to be comfortable.

“The oil or gel shot for the knee is a fluid that can be used to treat arthritis. Some people refer to it as a chicken shot. It's actually made out of rooster combs. The rooster comb can be used to produce a fluid that is similar to the fluid in the knee. When injected it can make the joint fluid a little thicker which help the joint feel better.

Something like using a heavier weight oil in a car motor. It might help rough surfaces glide by each other with less friction. "

He went on to explain that the product was expensive and was not superior to cortisone. The advertising was misleading. Cost wasn't a concern if the product worked better than a standard cortisone injection. The problem was that studies had found that the "gel shot" was no better than cortisone. Since it wasn't better, sometimes requiring up to five injections, and was ten times as expensive, it should be used as a backup option.

Molly did appreciate that Dr. Katz seemed patient and explained his approach to her and Homer. She also was impressed that he based his treatments on those that were supported by medical studies, and not ones that were pushed by drug companies. " This was commonly referred to as evidence-based medicine. It was considered a gold standard of treatment.

Dr. Katz added, "I know that everyone will be giving you advice on how to treat your knee. If you hear or read about something that I haven't covered or find a treatment that intrigues you, write it down and ask me at our next visit. There are lots of ways of treating arthritis that I'm happy to discuss with you . There are many websites and magazines that talk about treatments which exist only to make money for the companies that push the product. So, I encourage you to read and explore all options as much as you want. But try to understand there is a lot of hype regarding treatments. Please feel free to ask me for my thoughts and opinions on any new approaches to this condition."

Dr. Katz then opened the door and directed his assistance to help Molly and Homer to set up a therapy visit. He also said they should see him again in 4 weeks to assess the progress. If there were any problems with the medicine or if the knee didn't show some improvement in the next several days, Molly should call.

Homer and Molly, now not needing crutches, (her knee did feel great), walked out and made the next doctor visit and one for physical therapy. "Maybe things will be OK," Molly said in a hopeful voice to Homer.

Chapter 8

Medicine and Therapy

Between draining the knee, the injection, and a new prescription arthritis medicine,(she was given Celebrex and was told it wasn't better than Naprosyn, but maybe easier on her stomach), Molly was walking and doing most of her activities without a limp. There was still some soreness along the inside of her knee, just below the kneecap. The doctor had said that was where the joint line was arthritic. She didn't care what the reason was , as long as it felt better.

Therapy had been scheduled for three days after the injection. This would give the knee a chance to calm down if there was a reaction to the shot.

Molly showed up, registered, and sat in an area surrounded by other patients. Many had long incisions that were in various stages of healing. She tried not to stare. She peeked up as the patients with the long incisions limped back for their rehabilitation appointment. Some looked quite pleased with their progress. Others, obviously from recent surgery, did not look so happy with life. Molly heard her name called and went back to the therapy area. It was a clean and modern area with 12 different exam tables. It was well lit and two large 48-inch TVs were mounted in the corners. They were both playing cable shows. One had a cooking channel and the other was showing a house renovation program. Both had the sound turned off. The closed caption on the bottom of the screens let anyone interested to stay involved.

She was met by a therapist named Emily. About Molly's height, looking thin and energetic, she had her brown hair pulled back in a ponytail. She appeared to be in her 20's. "Great to meet you, " Emily said with bubbly enthusiasm. "Have a seat on the table and let's see what we can do to help you out."

Molly internally wondered why all medical persons referred to themselves as "we". She was always amused that in health care people always noted that "we" will help. They rarely referred to themselves as "I".

Emily asked Molly a few questions. There was a quick interview where Emily asked questions about her physical status, her lifestyle, what her goals were. Emily then went through the previous notes from the first visit with the doctor and asked Molly if the information was correct. "So, they drained and injected your knee," Emily stated, reading from the chart. "How's it feeling now?"

“Great!” Molly wanted this therapy stuff to be quick and short. Her knee had improved and her attitude was not to overly complicate her recovery with too many therapy visits. Molly had quietly felt that the therapy would be a waste of time. Something that was required by the insurance companies for them to pay the medical bills.

After a few minutes, her attitude had completely changed. Emily’s enthusiasm and attitude were infectious. She assured Molly that nothing would be done that would hurt or flare up her knee. Emily was going to work with Molly to get her knee stronger. That would allow recovery from this injury and help prevent any future injury.

The exercises that Molly was given were ones she could do at the gym. It wasn’t necessary to come to therapy to do exercises. Molly would be told how to do them and allowed to do them on her own. Follow up visits were simply to confirm progress or change exercises if pain occurs. A quick recovery was the plan. Do the exercises, get back into shape, get off the medications. Then, everything is back to normal.

With a well-defined home exercise plan, Molly left with an enthusiastic mindset. She was determined to follow the exercise protocol outlined by Emily. Molly was going to get better! All was progressing as hoped. The pain was less, the swelling was gone, and Molly was approaching her exercises with optimism.

She was at the gym every other day and performing the strengthening as instructed. She was avoiding that knee extension machine that caused pain. Working the muscles with leg raises rubber bands and ankle weights, her knee didn't hurt and the muscles seemed to be coming back to normal.

Unfortunately, the improvement lasted only 10 days. Just a little over two weeks from her first visit with the doctor, Molly was walking the dogs, all happily wagging their tails and straining their leashes. She stretched her left leg out to step down from the sidewalk curb. On placing weight on her leg, the pain was exquisite and took her breath away. It made her knee buckle and she almost fell, catching herself at the last moment putting all her weight on her right leg. Sensing a problem, Katy, the oldest dog stopped and turned to Molly, sensing something was wrong. “Ok guys, time to go home. Let’s not rush it,” Molly spoke to them like they could understand her words. Thankfully they were not that far from home.

Chapter 9

Back To the Doctor

Hobbling and limping home, Molly opened the door and collapsed on the couch. The dogs, suddenly sensing freedom, scooted upstairs to jump on the bed of her daughter Abby’s room.

Molly rubbed her knee, It was aching, sore, stiff, painful, and like a toothache, it wouldn’t stop hurting. Getting up with some difficulty, she limped to the kitchen and filled a bag with ice from the freezer. She had already taken her arthritis medicine from the Doctor. She grabbed two acetaminophen. She was told she might take acetaminophen for increased pain and it shouldn't interact with the arthritis medicine. She thought, "anything to help the pain."

Molly lay down on the couch and put the ice on her knee. Gulping the pills with a bottle of water, she considered a glass of wine, but her stomach was churning. She had been warned the arthritis pills could cause stomach ulcers and adding wine would increase that risk. Her stomach was already sensitive from all the medicines she had taken prior to the injection in the knee.

Her knee was incredibly sore. With a pillow under her knee and ice on top, she turned on the TV and tried to rest. Just as she was about to doze off, Homer opened the door and saw her predicament. Molly sat up and explained to Homer what had happened. A little misstep and now she was miserable. As she swung her knee over the edge of the couch to sit up, she gasped and saw that her knee was now huge. After the injection, the therapy, and the cortisone shot, everything looked great. Now, it looked worse than ever. "I think I should see the Doctor again, " Molly announced.

Homer looked at her and her knee and picked up the phone. Homer called and patiently went through the digital prompts and then the announcement that they should go to the emergency room if the condition was serious. Following the voice prompts for billing, therapy, the front desk, a prescription refill, and one of the four different physicians, Homer punched in the option for Dr. Katz. He was connected to a scheduling person.

Explaining the situation, he was put on hold for about five minutes. The receptionist than picked up. After apologizing for the delay, she said she had spoken to the assistant for Dr. Katz, They did have an opening in two days. There were no openings at all for today and Dr. Katz was in surgery the next day. She offered a different doctor or the emergency room for serious issues. After a quick conference with Molly while Homer held the phone against his chest, it was decided to take the appointment in two days. Molly preferred to see Dr. Katz who she felt understood his condition better than a new doctor. The knee was painful and swollen but ,Molly noted, "I'm not dying."

However, she was in pain and wondered if something could be given short term for pain and rest at night. Taking more arthritis medicine was not an option as her stomach was still churning. Homer asked the receptionist about something for the pain. He was concerned that the pain would be worse at night. His call was transferred to the assistant for Dr. Katz who picked up after another five minutes. Homer once again explained the situation and his concern about nighttime pain.

In the past, when Homer had a painful back issue, his physician had called in almost 50 Vicodin to help until the appointment that was scheduled in three days. Homer had only used four of them and ended up taking the rest back to the pharmacy to be destroyed. He had been surprised at how easily it was to get the painkillers.

Dr. Katz's medical assistant, Katy, told Homer that things had changed and new restrictions had been put in place on all pain medicine. Katy explained that no more than 2-3 days of pain medicine could be given and the amount would be limited and would not be refilled under any situation. She also said that a prescription could be called in only once. Any more medicine would require a prescription that was obtained from the physician.

Considering the current problems with narcotic drug use, Homer appreciated the new precautions. He said a few pills for nighttime pain would be more than adequate. Molly looked stoic, unhappy, and uncomfortable. After giving a pharmacy number, he was told that six pills would be called in. This was quite a different response from his past experience when asking for pain medicine. It was a welcome change considering the overuse of narcotics.

That evening, with Molly still on the couch, she took the pain medicine to see if it would help her rest and sleep. "These pills just make me feel stupid and tired," Molly complained as she finally went to sleep. Homer covered her with a blanket and one of the dogs, Katy, or Janey, jumped on her lap. Homer had trouble telling the dogs apart. They were all black, small, energetic, and loving.

The following day Molly got up and used the crutches. She hobbled around the house announcing to work that she was homebound till the next few days. Homer took Abby to school and helped out as best he could. Having him working at home was certainly helpful at times like this. Another evening of discomfort and it was time for the Doctor's visit. Molly had never been so happy to keep an appointment to see a doctor. The last two days she had been feeling useless. She couldn't walk the dogs, do the necessary shopping, help Abby or even go outside to get the mail. Suddenly she was aware of what it was like to be unable to move about comfortably and without pain.

Arriving at the front door of the office, Homer stopped the car and let her out. He parked the car and met her in the lobby. After a short wait, they were escorted back to the exam room they had been in the first time. Tiffany walked in, took Molly's blood pressure and updated the medical records. She looked at the shorts that Molly wore. She commented that it was good that she remembered to bring them. The paper examination shorts that they used for patients who needed them were ill fitting, wouldn't close, and were atrocious.

Tiffany closed the door behind her and said it wouldn’t be too much of a wait. Homer and Molly talked about random and mundane topics while waiting. Nothing serious. Anything to take Molly’s mind off of her worries about her knee. Homer was trying to be a good support person. Still, he was struggling to keep up the small talk. Molly saw he was worried. She appreciated that he was working hard to make her believe everything would be fine. Unfortunately, the pain and swelling in the knee was hard to ignore.

“Wow,” Dr. Katz observed as he walked in the room and looked at Molly’s knee, “That looks painful.” He walked over to Molly and placed his hand on her knee.

After feeling and squeezing the fluid in her knee and gently bending it, he ran his fingers along the sides of the knee. “Is the pain worse here, or here” as he moved his finger from the inner aspect of the knee below the kneecap and then to the top of her knee cap. Molly pointed to the inside aspect of her knee. Dr. Katz remarked that this was the joint line where the arthritis was occurring on the x-ray. Her whole knee ached. That area on the inner knee was the worst. Also, with the swelling, she had trouble bending her knee and there was pain in the back of her leg. She said the back was getting more uncomfortable and with the swelling, she couldn't get her knee to bend and get in the car without problems.

After reviewing the medical records and prior treatments, Dr. Katz sat down to discuss the situation. He said more cortisone should not be given. The last injection was recently done and repeating it would potentially cause added damage to the joint. He cautioned that in the past, physicians gave cortisone too frequently and may have accelerated joint injury. He did want to drain her knee. That would help her pain. He recommended the gel or chicken shot that they discussed during the first visit. Since the cortisone had apparently not provided long term relief, it was worth trying a different product. Although the gel shot was not necessarily better than cortisone, it was different and it was worth trying to see if she would have a longer benefit.

Dr. Katz also said it was time for an MRI. The failure to improvement with medicine, therapy and a cortisone injection warranted a more detailed evaluation of the knee.

Draining the knee was just like before. Some freezing medicine, the numbing shot, and the fluid was removed. Dr. Katz said the product he injected only required a single shot. Some of the gel injections required up to five visits.

The shots required insurance authorization due to expense. While Molly had been waiting in the exam room, the office had called and received approval to give the injection.

Injecting the syringe of thick honey colored fluid didn't hurt. The amount of the amber yellow jelly being injected was about 4 tablespoons.

"How will this help the pain in the back of her knee? The fluid you took out was from the front of the knee and the injection is in the front," Homer pointed out to Dr. Katz.

"Good question! How does the fluid in the front cause the swelling in the back of the knee? Have you ever heard about a Baker's cyst?" Dr. Katz inquired to both Homer and Molly.

Dr. Katz answered his own question. "Well, it has nothing to do with the job or occupation of being a baker. It was first described by a Professor William Baker, in England, in 1877. He found that patients with disease in the knee had swelling in the front and back of the knee. To help the pain Dr. Baker did surgery and removed the cyst in the back. And, removing the cyst in the back, (which Homer realized was being done 30 years before the use of modern anaesthesia) did not work. The cyst and the pain in the back always recurred. This was because the fluid in the back flows from the front. So, Dr. Baker realized that to get rid of the back cyst, you must cure the problem causing fluid in the front of the knee. This cyst was named after the physician who described it and the futility of removing it."

"Hopefully, the gel shot will work and calm the knee down. This will prevent the fluid in the front from coming back. And, if the fluid doesn't come back, the pain in the back and the stiffness will be gone."

Once again, the knee felt better after removal of the fluid. Molly got up and headed to the door. The assistant sat at her desk and asked Molly where she wanted to do the MRI. There was a facility closer to home which Molly chose. After a phone call to the insurance company, the MRI was authorized and scheduled.

Chapter 10

After the MRI, Now what?

Molly drove herself to the MRI facility. Having the MRI performed was easy. Molly cheerfully told the technician that she had no fear of enclosed places or claustrophobia. The machine used was "open" and only her knee was place in the tube. After some positioning and setup, the imaging was quickly performed.

After a little wait, Molly was given a USB stick which contained a digital copy of the imaging. She was told to wait for a call to review the findings from her doctor. The call from Dr. Katz's office came the next day.

Katy, his assistant, gave Molly some basic information about the findings. There was arthritis and it was called grade 4. That was the worst level with grade 0 being a knee without any damage. Dr. Katz needed to speak to her and review the imaging.

An appointment was made for the next day.

Limping into the office, Molly sat with Homer in the waiting room with Homer providing hopeful banter. Molly not so subtly ignored him dreading the results of the MRI. She knew it showed arthritis, which was seen on the x-rays. There had to be additional damage that the x-ray missed. She wanted to know why the shot didn't help.

After going into the exam room, the assistant pulled the MRI imaging onto a computer display screen. Molly and Homer waited in the room staring at the black and white shadows that looked like alien drawings. Or, Molly thought, like a Rorschach test. She was about to say the top image looked like a sinister villain when Dr. Katz walked in. "Well, let's see what we have," he muttered without saying hello.

He turned to the screen and quickly scanned through what appeared to be about 100 images. "Haven't you read the report?" Molly asked him. She assumed that the report was important and his looking at the films would add little to figuring out what was wrong with her knee.

"I always read the report. Radiologists look at the MRI but don't understand all the clinical symptoms and objective findings. It is important to correlate the specific complaints and issues with the MRI. There are a lot of findings on an MRI that may be of no consequence. A small meniscus tear that isn't in an area of pain may be interesting, but not important to the treatment. And, if surgery is needed, I need to see bone structure, alignment, and geometry. These are things the official reading may not reveal." Dr. Katz said this without turning around, talking to the screen.

After a few moments, he turned to her. He quickly examined the knee and checked the swelling and areas of pain. Her knee was still bent from the fluid that had reaccumulated and was stiff. "The MRI confirms the injury and diagnosis. Your knee has severe arthritis. This is what the x-rays revealed and is seen clearly on the MRI." Dr. Katz told her, "You have rather severe arthritis with loss of the cartilage that lines the joint. There is almost complete joint line collapse and the bone has developed cysts of fluid from the loss or cartilage. This causes the bone to weaken and results in further joint damage. Because of all the problems with the bone and cartilage, the meniscus has shredded and is no longer functioning. "

He added, "There is evidence of bone edema. That is inflammation and vascular changes in the actual bone of the knee. It's like a bruise of the bone. That can cause pain, discomfort and weakness in the strength of the bone. This may allow the bone to collapse."

Molly was both happy, sad and shocked at hearing the news. She was glad that there was a reason for all the pain. She wasn't imagining or complaining without a reason. But the reality that her knee was in such bad shape was disturbing. Looking straight at Dr. Katz she asked him what her options were. "Considering the x-rays, your MRI, and the failure to improve with steroids and therapy, you have limited options. You can limp and have pain, realizing this probably will get worse, try a brace for short term benefits, or have surgery. Based on everything that has happened to date, you are going to need surgery. And, if you decide on surgery, then a knee replacement will be needed" Dr. Katz said. He looked straight at her eyes while he told her the need for an operation in order to sense her reaction.

Molly exclaimed, "I’m too young. That's not possible...there must be an easier option." She looked at Homer for support. "I have friends who have had outpatient arthroscopy. That just requires a band aid and crutches for a day. And what about stem cells?" She blurted out every treatment option she had every heard of in desperation.

Hoisting up onto the edge of desk, Dr. Katz leaned back. He slowly and calmly said, "Let's look at the facts and go through every option." He then explained everything.

Chapter 11

Options Before Surgery

Molly listened while Dr. Katz explained the condition and the approaches that might give her relief from her pain. She learned that certain cells in the human body could not regenerate, heal or regrow when damaged. These cells included brain cells, certain cells in your eye, and, of importance to her, cartilage cells. Once damaged, cartilage cells die. When they die, they slowly disappear and the protective covering to the bone that they provide is gone. The bone is then exposed. That is the pathology in arthritis. When rough bone surfaces rub against each other during joint motion, it hurts, grinds, and has resultant swelling.

There are non-operative treatments or non-surgical approaches. Some approaches such as TNS or transcutaneous nerve stimulation might help pain but will not improve the overall condition. Other options such as braces and ultrasound might give some improvement, but the cartilage damage will get worse over time. None of these options delayed or stopped the progression of the disease.

"What about supplements? I've heard about things such as glucosamine and something called chondroitin sulfate. My dogs take that and it seems to help their joint pain," Molly offered as a treatment option.

Dr. Katz explained that those supplements seem to work more in dogs than in people. There certainly was no reason not to try them.

How they were supposed to work was unclear. He explained that cartilage cells were like pillows stuffed with gelatin. These gelatin filled cells looked like water balloons and provided the cushion over the bone. In arthritis, the cells died and the gelatin leaked out and disappeared. The collapsed cells have no gelatin and there is no longer a cushion. By taking products that the gelatin is made of, glucosamine and chondroitin, they could be absorbed by the cells and the gelatin might not disappear after injury.

However, there is little science to show this actually works and the cartilage cells don't seem to make new gelatin after injury. Many studies show taking glucosamine or chondroitin is better than a placebo in humans.

Additionally, once the cells are gone, as in Molly's case, there are no cells left to make the cushion. "It's like using a product to keep you from losing your hair after all the hair is gone", Dr. Katz remarked. "Once your bald, the products won't work. And, in your case, the cartilage cells are gone. "

Dr. Katz then proceeded to give her a detailed update on current treatments. She listened attentively and learned quite a bit. It was certainly different than the newspaper headlines that she had read regarding how to treat arthritis.

Stem cells, the hope and future for many conditions, has been tried in knee arthritis. Cartilage stem cells grown in cultures and transplanted in the knee have been shown to work in some conditions. But the use of these cells in generalized knee arthritis has never been shown to be effective. Dr. Katz explained that simply injecting cells in the knee didn't result in the cells attaching and growing. The cells needed an appropriate environment. In arthritis, the underlying bone and vascular supply is diseased. The cells injected would not stick and start to make a new surface. Such cell therapy did work in specific cases, but not for diffused arthritis.

It would be like trying to cure diabetes by injecting insulin making pancreatic cells into a person. Just putting cells into a joint or the body does not make a new organ or joint surface. In young people, with extremely limited areas of damage surrounded by normal joint surface, such cell transplants can work. However, in osteoarthritis, the entire area is damaged.

Imagine performing a hair plug to a small area of baldness in the middle of a head of healthy hair. Then consider a hair plug to someone who has a completely bald head. In osteoarthritis, the knee has lost all the normal cartilage cells. Essentially, the knee is completely bald. A transplant won't work.

There are some other injections such as plasma rich protein. This is where blood is taken from the person a specific cells are removed from the blood and injected into the knee. These cells are thought to act like stem cells and also decrease inflammation.

Some studies show that injecting PRP or plasma rich protein helps knee pain. It is similar to the gel shot or cortisone for pain relief. It might last longer than the other injections, but PRP did not make cartilage regrow. It was a good treatment to try to delay surgery. But ultimately surgery would be needed for bad arthritis.

Other procedures, such as breaking the lower leg and realigning the bone did provide improvement for certain forms of arthritis. By making the boney alignment different, the area of damage was protected from the full weight of the limb. It was similar to walking on the side of the foot to avoid a painful arch.

This realignment approach required a slow recovery and had unpredictable recovery results for certain persons. Molly was told that the surgery worked best in taller persons with bowed legs. Having a knee that was not bowed made her a poor candidate for this technique called a high tibial osteotomy.

She was also told that such a realignment of the lower leg for arthritis had certain risks such as the bone not healing. And this risk was greater in females. Plus, the leg realignment did not stop the arthritis from getting worse. And a total knee after the high tibial osteotomy might not do as well.

Arthroscopy for her knee would provide no benefit or help. The doctor stated many peer reviewed and published papers that had shown arthroscopy for knee arthritis was no more effective than an injection. There was only short-term improvement. It had been shown that therapy without surgery had fewer complications and, in some cases, better improvement. Placebo surgery, one where small holes in the knee were made but no surgery was performed, had as good a result as when surgery had been performed for the arthritis.

It was now almost universally accepted that arthroscopy was of limited if any benefit and provided only short-term relief. Dr. Katz opened a patient education pamphlet, leaned forward, and pointed to the title, "Knee Replacement Surgery". Then, opening the pamphlet that showed a shiny metal device. He explained that this was her best option.

Chapter 12

Time to Consider a Knee Replacement

"Total knees are not a simple hinge that replaces the knee joint. Think of them more like surface replacements. Your bones and ligaments are almost entirely preserved. They are not removed. All that is replaced are the damaged coatings of the bone. It would be like having a new Teflon surface being put on a damaged pan." Molly listened while Dr. Katz continued. "The modern knee replacement resurfaces all the bone with a metal and plastic surface that replaces the damaged cartilage. The shiny metal glides on the plastic like an ice skate on ice. There is almost no friction and the knee uses your own bone and ligaments for the basic framework."

While imagining the artificial knee, Molly envisioned a giant metal robotic type device in her small body. "How are you ever going to get it to fit my small leg?"

Dr. Katz responded "There is not just one size. There are systems that measure your knee and determine what is the correct size. The knees come in over 10 sizes for the femur, 10 sizes for the tibia and plastic blocks in many thicknesses that act as sizing shims. They can be mixed and matched to fit almost any person. They come small enough to fit a child and large enough for the tallest basketball player. Every size and every possible combination are always ready for use."

"How about just a partial knee? I've heard you can just replace the damaged part. Isn't that easier?" Molly whispered.

Dr. Katz looked up from the pamphlet. "Unfortunately, I cannot recommend that. Your knee has damage on multiple areas and is widespread. A partial knee only fixes one small part of a knee. It works only if the damage is isolated to one area. If all areas are not fixed, the damaged parts will continue to deteriorate and cause significant pain and swelling. Ultimately, another knee surgery would be needed. A full knee surgery will provide treatment to all areas of damage."

It appeared that Molly was going to need a new knee. She had not improved with rest, injections or therapy. Medications had not helped and the MRI showed complete loss of cartilage with joint line collapse in multiple areas. She had pain, swelling and instability. Her lifestyle was affected and she needed a cane to walk without falling. It was time for a new knee.

Chapter 13

Picking the Perfect Knee

After hearing and absorbing what her orthopedic specialist had told her, Molly and Homer left the office to discuss it over. She was told by Dr. Katz that there was no rush, but there were limited options until surgery was performed. She got out of the car, using her cane due to pain, and sat down at the computer to do research on knee replacements. She was determined to become a total knee expert.

After typing "total knee replacement" into Google, she found the first dozen responses were from lawyers advertising services for malpractice. After refining the search to those involving "total knee best results", she got the same responses.

She rapidly learned that there was far too much information on the internet, far too many lawyers, and too many personal blogs to do random searches. It seemed everyone who had a knee replacement had posted a video or had a web site with personal opinions that were not based on any science or fact. She would need guidance.

A friend and physician recommended she restrict her search to the online publication site PubMed. This was a database established by the National Institute of Health. It contained only peer reviewed online publications in the field of medicine. It was considered the database of knowledge for physicians seeking top quality papers on any topic.

Also, it was suggested that she look at information that was provided by medical societies. She found a fair amount of easy to read and unbiased information from the American Academy of Orthopaedic Surgeons. After reviewing and absorbing as much information as possible, Molly made a list of topics for her next visit with Dr. Katz.

She needed more information on each of these areas of knee surgery. It seemed that these specific issues could affect the outcome and success of the operation.

They were:

1.) Computer surgery.
2.) Patient specific instruments.
3.) Gender specific knee.
4.) Allergies to knee replacements.
5.) Using cement in the knee.
6.) Knees with mobile bearings.
7.) Different types and manufacturers and results.

Her head was stuffed with ideas, questions and concerns when she next showed up to talk to Dr. Katz. She was prepared for the visit. Dr. Katz walked into the exam room and Molly took out here clipboard with questions. Rather than being put off, Dr. Katz thanked her for bringing the questions in writing.

Dr. Katz took the papers and proceeded to explain each issue and wrote down comments to each area of concern. On returning home, she summarized each issue and incorporated the information from Dr. Katz. She typed the information into her computer and printed out the results. When finished, she showed it to Homer.

Computer surgery

Computer surgery involves robotic systems. The robots have mechanical arms that are partially controlled by computers and the surgeon who assists in guiding the cutting drills and saws. Before surgery is performed, images of the knee are downloaded into the computer. This allows the computer to understand the anatomy of the knee.

Some of the robotic devices get added information by having the surgeon mark certain areas of the knee with a probe that can be sensed by the computer. This gives the computer the necessary information to do the surgery.

All of the computer or robotic systems are designed so that the surgeon can control the cutting devices. This prevents any possible error from the computer. This correction is done if there is a need for minor correction.

The results of this type of surgery are good. It does involve additional imaging, equipment and time to perform the surgery.

However, robotic surgery has not been shown to improve outcomes or final results. There is little evidence to show it is superior to a good surgeon. Results of this type of approach have not been shown to be better.

It does require use of a specific implant device to work with the robot and computer. Each computer system is specific for only one manufacturer. So, you have limited implant options.

Due to added hospital costs, added imaging, limited implant use, and lack of evidence of improved results, it is not accepted as better. It is merely different.

Patient specific instruments

Like computer or robotic surgery, this involves instruments designed off of pre-operative imaging that assists in the insertion and implanting of the new knee. They have nothing to do with a custom knee. They are used to help make the cuts for a standard knee. These specific insertion instruments are designed for a specific person and only used once.

The use of these patient specific insertion instruments has been shown to give good results. However, many studies have shown the instruments do not give better outcomes. Due to added costs and imaging, the systems are not always used and have not been accepted as being better than traditional surgery.

It is commonly thought that the custom instruments mean that there is a custom implant. This is not the case. The implants are the same whether the instruments used to insert the implants are patient specific or standard. The end result is that the same standard knee is used in each case.

Patient specific instruments are becoming popular for the reason that they may make the surgical procedure faster. By not having to assemble jigs and use alignment rods, the surgery is faster. This is an advantage.

Gender specific Knees

This was an advertising gimmick by a company interested in increasing the use of their knee. Many research papers have shown that with the many sizing options available for all knee implants, the gender specific knee is identical to the standard knee. In fact, the results of the gender specific knee were in some ways inferior to the traditional knee due to design issues. It is no longer being advertised and companies no longer describe a knee that is based on gender.

Allergies to knee implants

This is an interesting area of ongoing research. Most artificial knees are made from stainless steel. It is accepted that some people do have allergies to the metals in the knee. This may be a cause for pain and discomfort after a knee replacement. If there is a history of metal sensitivity, allergy testing may be needed.

Some knees have ceramic coatings to try to avoid the allergic condition. Some knees are titanium However, true metal allergy is rare and if there is no prior history of metal contact dermatitis, the risk is exceedingly low.

Blood testing is not a reliable method of finding metal allergies. If there is a concern, an allergy specialist may do skin testing or perform a very specific analysis of white cells for sensitivity to certain metals.

Ceramic coated is sometimes used to prevent metal allergies. This "hides and covers" the metal. It is not used in all knees as the coating process is complex, time consuming, and limits the design options. At one point there was a concern the coating might flake off.

The vast majority of total knees are made of standard polished metal which is similar to stainless steel. There is limited evidence that ceramic coated knees or titanium knees last longer or have any benefit except in metal allergy conditions.

Cemented or non-cemented knee

There are different methods used to get the metal components to "stick" to the bone. One of the more common reasons for a knee replacement to fail or not work is the loosening of the implant to the bone. If there is not a solid union between the underlying bone structure and the implant, then there will be recurrent pain and swelling. This is because the knee is loose. Cement is used, but it is not a glue. It is a substance that acts like mortar between bricks. It flows into crevices in the bone and the implant and provides a bond that is based on the strength of how the cement grip to the rough interface areas.

The weak link is that the cement may fail or the grip on the bone may deteriorate over time. Like a crown on a tooth, it may not last forever.

One advantage of cement is that it is instantly hard and set at the end of surgery. Cement is ready to take the full weight of the body the moment the surgery is over. It should last 20-30 years. Also, if there is a chance of an infection, antibiotics can be added to the cement. This provides increased protection from an infection.

If cement is not used, a special type of implant, commonly referred to as porous or bony ingrowth is used. When using a non-cemented knee, the underlying bone will literally grow into the knee. This might appear better as it doesn't include the addition of a foreign substance like cement. However, ingrowth into the knee is not predictable and sometimes is spotty or may not occur. In these cases, the condition known as fibrous ingrowth occurs. Scar tissue, not bone grows into the knee. This is too weak to last and the knee will fail. When boney ingrowth occurs, it may take months to become solid. This may require a delay in weight bearing.

Overall, there is no apparent advantage or disadvantage of using or not using cement. However, due to the decades of experience, the immediate weight bearing potential and possible use of antibiotics, the cemented knee is the more popular choice at this time.

Knees with mobile bearings

Total knees are complex reproductions of the actual knee. They are not exact models of the knee. An implant duplicates the normal knee in motion but does not duplicate the specific multiple parts of the knee. There are no menisci, the anterior and/or posterior cruciates may be removed, and the multiple small ligaments that control meniscus motion are sacrificed in the surgery.

An artificial knee duplicates the complexity of a normal knee by inserting a polyethylene or plastic part between the two metal surfaces. This piece of plastic is molded and designed to reproduce and mimic the actions of the many tissues that are removed. It is a marvel of engineering. And it does a fantastic job. However, it is not as good as what nature gave us.

In order to allow a more "natural" feeling joint, a number of engineers have developed different models and designs that might mimic the actions of the meniscus and ligaments. Some of these designs allowed the plastic insert to rotate on a central pivot or bearing. These are called mobile bearing knees. It was thought this might give additional motion and make the joint feel like a real knee, (which has a certain amount of rotation).

It turns out that people can't tell the difference between knees that have mobile bearings or ones that are fixed. There appears to be no significant difference when comparing mobile knees to those with static joints or non-mobile bearings. There are theoretical advantages of each but there is no proven superiority of one over the other.

Which is the best knee?

Molly summarized all of the information into a simple conclusion. It appeared that despite different techniques of insertion, computers, robots, bearings, metals and design, they all had good and bad results.

Large review studies have found that there is little difference in results. Some knee designs have known issues, such as early wear, but the reasons for the problems have been figured out and those designs are no longer used. With each new generation of knee replacements, new concepts are tried and utilized in the hope of providing a better and longer lasting knee. Some of these changes are found to have early complications and they are rapidly removed from the marketplace.

The overwhelming decision regarding what knee to use is based more on the surgeon's familiarity with the system design and familiarity with potential complications than with any advertising hype.

Essentially, all modern knees have reproducible and good results.

Chapter 14

Making a Decision

Molly read her pamphlets, asked friends, looked on the internet, and found that everyone had an opinion about which was the best knee. After reviewing all the information, it was apparent that there were good and bad results with all knee surgeries. And the results seemed to be remarkably similar regardless of the type of knee or the technique.

Review articles that compared specific types and manufacturers of knees found that there was little evidence that one knee was clearly superior. All knees could fail or give troubles and all knees had patients who loved the results. It didn't seem to matter if the knee was cementless, cemented, mobile, static or made of titanium.

There was only small differences in how the patients did. "Bad knees", those with bad designs, were no longer in use. Total knee replacements have been done for long enough that almost all the things that made knees fail early in the recovery had been figured out and were no longer used. Rigid hinged knees had lots of troubles, but they are not used in modern medicine. Some of the early plastics were brittle and failed. Those were removed from use over a decade ago. Having discovered what works, knees became more similar in design. They were based on the same established mechanical guidelines. Surgical preference was based on training and familiarity with a system.

It didn't matter if the knee surgery was performed by a robot, a computer, or a surgeon. What every paper and article found was that the technology had made the surgery reproducible. A skilled surgeon had results as good as the most advanced custom device or robotic system. The common denominator in any successful knee surgery was the skill of the surgeon. It's not the ingredients but the cook who knows how to get a good result. And a good surgeon will have predictably good results.

What did matter was experience. Not surprisingly, it was found that the more surgeries a physician did and the more surgeries the hospital performed, the better the short- and long-term outcomes. So, skill and knowledge trumped the fanciest designs and technology. Picking a good physician was the most important choice in the surgery.

Chapter 15

What to Expect

Ultimately the question to be answered is what can be expected from a total knee in a person who is active with a health family and lifestyle?

"That answer", Dr. Katz told Molly, "is still not fully understood. The results of knee replacements in elderly and less active persons are extremely good. Over 90% are pleased with the results with improvements in lifestyle. It is rare to have a more sedentary person with a complaint regarding his or her knee replacement. "

"As knee replacements got better and the longevity of the knee surgery improved, younger and younger persons opted for a replacement if there was debilitating pain. However, with younger patients came higher expectations."

"It used to be that simply walking was considered a sign of success. Young patients wanted to play tennis, jog, and ride a bike. With these increased needs came increasing dissatisfaction."

Molly understood that knee replacements now are expected to last at least 20 years and, in some cases, knees are doing well at 30 and 40 years. "However," Dr. Katz told her, "as younger and more active patients were getting surgery, there is a concern that the knee would wear out earlier due to the stresses on the joint. This leads to the finding that satisfaction in younger persons is dropping and is only around 80%.

And, if there is continued pain, it is often impossible to find the reason for the discomfort that persisted after surgery. "

What this meant, Molly realized, is that surgery could provide a great benefit. A full relief of pain, swelling and a return to near normal activity. But there was no guarantee. Dr. Katz did say that he had patients who jogged and played tennis. However, these patients are not the norm and were at risk for earlier failure or problems with their knee. They did these higher level of activities in spite of the precautions given. They were called in the medical field, "outliers". Essentially, they were patients who exceeded expectations but could not be used as an example that others should follow.

Molly internally hoped that she might be an outlier. She was quite confident that her doctor was skilled and his credentials were excellent. The knee he preferred was a modern design with a proven track record.

"I don't want to be the first person to have a new knee design. I want one that has years of proven good results", Dr. Katz stated. Molly liked that approach. To her it was like buying a car. A simple Honda has been proven to work for millions of customers. The exotic custom designed Ferrari could be a maintenance nightmare. She wanted simple and proven designs that would last for decades.

Chapter 16

Planning for the future

It was time to proceed. Molly had made up her mind. She had scheduled the surgery with Dr. Katz and was preparing the time off to allow a full recovery. She understood that she needed at least 2 weeks to feel good. It would another 4 weeks until she was nearly independent regarding driving and activities. Three months might be necessary until she was nearly her old self with six months for full recovery.

She decided that the pain, swelling and limitations from her knee were too much of a limitation. To live with a lesser quality of life was not in her future. Aware of the risks, benefits and gains from surgery, she was ready for her new knee.

How the surgery went, the rehabilitation and complications, well that is a story in itself.

To be continued
......Molly has a Total Knee Replacement Surgery
and then
.... Molly has Complications from her Total Knee Surgery.

Printed in Great Britain
by Amazon

53570012R00063